Age with Audacious Confidence

21+ Tips to Look & Feel Younger

ALICIA COURI

Dedication

This book is dedicated to my parents Dr. Francis Davis and Lena Davis for blessing me with great genes.

Also to my beloved late Pastor Stan Sr. who taught me Psalm 103:5, which became one of my very favorite scriptures.

"Age with Audacious Confidence" is an un-put-downable guide to looking spectacular at any age. The tips that Alicia shares especially about running and make-up are outstanding. I shall smile away towards always looking younger with "Age younger" in my pocket."

~ Geetha Krishnan

Mom, Wife, International Best selling Author, Corporate Trainer, Radio show Host, Gratitude Leadership Coach, Certified Professional International Speaker, Philanthropist.

"There are a lot of people with various health issues and I would recommend them Mrs. Alicia's book to age younger and improve their health, figure, and features. All of her tips are every helpful and really make a difference to your life; the one I have to improve is eating foods and supplements since I am working on being a vegan. I may be a 20-year-old guy in college now, but after reading this book, I now know what to do when I am older and for now on."

~ Lew Sterling Jr.

Student, Miami, Florida

"If you're looking for the optimum way to elevate energy levels and improve your appearance, this is the most sensible approach for anyone to preserve youthfulness".

Leasha West

CEO, West Insurance and Financial Group, Inc

Alicia's refreshing style lights up these 21 tips that she shares from experience and from her heart. Both women and men benefit from her insight. . I've even shared Alicia's makeup techniques with my daughters!

~ Don Boehm

Anti-Aging Solutions

St Charles, Illinois

Table of Contents

Introduction .... - 1 -

#1 Watch Your thoughts and Words: Psalms 103:1-7 .... - 4 -

2 Mix it up .... - 7 -

#3 Remembering Your Youth .... - 9 -

#4 Becoming More of Who You Were Created To Be! .... - 11 -

#5 Posture – Good Posture & Aging .... - 14 -

#6 Take Good Care of Your Teeth .... - 17 -

#7 Smile Wider .... - 19 -

#8 LOL – Laugh Out Loud!!! .... - 22 -

#9 Stay Away From The Sun .... - 28 -

#10 Create a Daily Skin Care Routine .... - 32 -

#11 Run for your life .... - 37 -

#12 Rev up your metabolism .... - 42 -

#13 Clothes make the man/woman .... - 47 -

#14 Foods & Supplements that Build & Improve Collagen.............- 53 -

#15 Hair Cut &/ or Color ....- 56 -

#16 Take Care of Neck, Chest, Elbows and Hands. ....- 58 -

#17 Using Effective Makeup Techniques ....- 60 -

#18 Avoid Alcohol ....- 66 -

#19 – No Smoking ....- 68 -

#20 – Drink Lots of Water ....- 70 -

#21 – Love Yourself ....- 72 -

Bonus Tips.. - 76 -

Conclusion ....- 106 -

Resources ....- 108 -

Introduction

As a Beauty & Style expert, I am frequently asked about anti-aging products and treatments from my clients. As a 47 year old married woman with 3 children I am often times mistaken for a single woman in her 20's with no kids. The question I get asked the most is "What are you doing girl because I want some of that".

I had to really take some time to think about exactly what I was doing, and had done throughout my life because honestly, I had never really thought about it before. I just lived my life and chalked it up to genetics. But after overwhelming requests of, "What's your secret" I began thinking about how I've lived my life the last 20+ years and what the major contributors could have been that have me looking and feeling decades younger".

I didn't want this book to be all about diet and exercise, (although those are incredibly important elements in this process), because I am neither a slave to the gym nor to any particular diet plan. I eat a relatively healthy diet, I'm not into sweets so I don't eat desserts, chocolates or candy much, unless it's a very special occasion or on the off chance I have a particular craving, I'm also not a big snacker but I will eat popcorn at the movies or potato chips from time to time, and I do like me some Cheetos, but my preferred snacks are typically delicious fruits and vegetables.

With all that in mind, I have isolated at least 21 things I do, and have been doing, (and a couple helpful hints from additional research). Some of these I've done for most of my life and a few that I've adopted more recently. I'm sure as you read through this book there may be some things you yourself are doing and you might say to me, "Alicia really what's the big deal, I already do that" and that's what I thought but the cumulative effect of some of these things have had a tremendous impact in my life and will probably do the same for you.

Here we go!

#1 Watch Your thoughts and Words:

Psalms 103:1-7

One of my favorite scriptures in the Bible is found in Palms 103. The Psalmist says this: "He satisfies my mouth with good things, so that my youth is renewed like that of the Eagle". This stated as one of the great benefits of God's blessings.

So I have maintained for the most part very positive thoughts and words about myself, my body and my youth. I work at not thinking or speaking negatively about my body and I don't consider my age at all. I still see myself and feel like a teenager.

The truth that researchers and scientists are confirming is that your thoughts that manifest into words, not only alter the structure of your brain, but it also manifest in the body.

Dr. Caroline Leaf has done extensive studies over 20 years on how toxic or negative thoughts physically change the structure of your brain which in turn affects the body. Your thoughts can affect you whether good or bad.

In an incredible study in the 1960s on the effect of sound on physical objects, Dr. Hans Jenny placed sand, fluid and powders on metal plates, which he vibrated with a special frequency generator and a speaker. His experiments produced beautiful and intricate patterns that were unique to each individual vibration. It was interesting to note that these varying patterns remained intact as long as the sound pulsed through the substance. If the sound stopped, the pattern collapsed.

These experiments show that sound can indeed alter form, different frequencies produce different results, and sound actually creates and maintains form.

This should not be any surprise because in Genesis it gives an account of how the universe was framed:

And God said, let there be light: and there was light…

Everything God said in the beginning of creation was created. In addition when Man was created he created us in His own image and likeness, meaning; we create in the same manner as God did in the beginning.

Don't forget… As a man thinks in his heart, so is he…

So think and speak yourself young!

2 Mix it up

Don't stick to the same routine, your body & brain like challenges! Ok so there's lots of evidence out there that speak about the benefits of switching your routine. For me it came from never having worked a conventional job. I've been a Flight Attendant, a Stylist on photo and video shoots, a writer and for more than a decade an onsite professional Hair & Makeup Artist, a Speaker and an actor, in addition to being a wife and mother. My life is full of variety. Some think my life is crazy, I love that it's unpredictable. Now that doesn't mean if you work a 9-5 job that you can't find a way to challenge your everyday routine and mix it up.

When you exercise regularly, you are encouraged to switch up your routine because when you change your exercise or workout routine it challenges your muscles to work different strengths so you're not building the same muscles over and over again. For your brain the benefits are tremendous. It causes you to think in different ways. In her research, Dr. Caroline Leaf talks about building new neuropathways in your brain by changing your thinking especially in areas that are negative and don't allow you to grow. Just like a child who is constantly building these neuropathways through learning and growing, you can do the same and by doing so, it will help keep you younger.

So switch it up!

#3 Remembering Your Youth

Reliving the things you loved when you were younger. Ok don't judge me but one of my favorite shows in the early 90's was 'Married with Children" Al Bundy in every episode would talk about scoring 4 touch downs in a single game. Yes reliving the glory days can get old for those around you, but remembering things like how you fell in love, your first crush and many of the happier moments in your life brings joy to your heart and raises your endorphin levels.

In a study at Harvard University, people who were placed in an environment that resembled their youth—with movies, music, and memorabilia from the past—experienced marked improvements in their memory, vision, happiness level, and overall health. Lead researcher Dr. Ellen Langer of the Mindfulness Institute said, "It shows that our mind-set is what limits us".

Here's a great exercise you can do for yourself, put together a playlist from the best years of your life, spend a few hours just immersed in the sights and sounds of the past and allow the happy memories to flood you. Remember where you were and how you felt when you heard a particular song. Also revisit your goals, dreams and aspirations. It's never too late!

So do something that really takes you back to a happier

place!

#4 Becoming More of Who You Were Created To Be!

"There is no greater thing you can do with your life, and your work than follow your passions in a way that serves the world and you"

~ Sir Richard Branson

There is a light that emanates from within you when you discover what you were put on this earth to do, and that life brings you so much joy and youthfulness. Look at women like Suzanne Sommers, Marilu Henner, Tina Turner, Iman, JLo, all living their lives with passion and a purpose that extend far beyond themselves. I have noticed the more I step into my own purpose and passion, I have more radiance that goes far beyond just the way I look. I am more energetic, more productive and have more fire to get things done. This discovery came after a couple years of personal growth coaching that really helped me connect to the person I was meant to be, in addition to my years of spiritual growth - getting closer to God and discovering more of Him in me.

Often times things about us are labeled as bad or wrong or as flaws and weaknesses, when in fact they can be gifts and talents that are just misappropriated. For instance you may have been labeled as a problem student that talked too much in class – when in fact you were practicing to be an epic talk show host. Or maybe you were labeled the dreamer or class clown but that dreamer turned into a visionary CEO and a Comedian. A hammer can be used as a tool to build or one that destroys, it has the capability for both it all depends on how you choose to use it.

A couple resources for you that would help you discover more of yourself. If you have never taken the Kolbe A test, that measures your conative or your instinctive modes of operation. It is how you were wired. This test helped me so so much because there are no judgements, only shows you how to best utilize the way to naturally approach tasks and life. Briggs Myers test is a way to find your strengths, these can change and you can build new strengths but this helps give you a benchmark. As an entrepreneur, Wealth Dynamics is another test you can take that measures you fastest and easiest path to wealth and hat suits your particular personality.

So work diligently at becoming more of who you were created to be!

#5 Posture – Good Posture & Aging

I truly dislike seeing women slouch, it's so unhealthy and it is not a youthful posture. It makes you look older. When I was a Flight Attendant one of the exercises in our training dealt with proper posture, we all had to learn to walk tall. Even as far back as the 2nd grade, I remember my teacher urging us to always have our shoulders up and back and our necks elongated. Correct posture helps you breathe so much deeper and easier and allows more oxygen which helps blood circulation, which in turn improves your youth.

Research shows that poor posture extracts a high price as you age because:

- It can limit your range of motion.

- Muscles can be permanently shortened or stretched when a slumped over position becomes your normal position.

- Muscles and ligaments that have been shortened or stretched no longer function as they should.

- Poor posture can make you look older than you are.

When you are slumped over, hunched over, or not standing straight, you can add years to your appearance. A damaging contributor to poor posture is cell phone use. So be aware of how much you slouch when using your phones.

For women, the more rounded the shoulders, the more breasts may sag. Any woman, no matter what her age, can help reduce the sag in her breasts by nearly 50% by simply standing tall.

Here are a few tips on improving your posture when standing or sitting.

- Hold your head high

- Position your chin firmly forward

- Have your shoulders back

- Stick your chest out

- Have your stomach tucked in to increase your balance.

So stand up straight and tall!

#6 Take Good Care of Your Teeth

Hopefully I don't have to tell you to brush regularly, because good oral health is key to looking younger or can make you look older. Coffee, red wine, and other foods can stain teeth over time, and having yellow teeth can age you. However I personally have sensitive teeth so I don't use teeth whiteners but I do use whitening toothpaste from time to time. Using hydrogen peroxide with baking soda, Coconut oil pulling or activated charcoal have all been proven as natural whitening alternatives to those whitening trays especially if you have sensitive teeth. Flossing daily also helps healthy teeth and gums. I always carry floss with me and floss every single day. One of my best tricks to make my teeth look even whiter is to wear bright colored lipstick.

Red is my favorite!

So brush and floss for a whiter smile!

#7 Smile Wider

Smiling was always a challenge for me for many years. I was so self-conscious about it, especially in pictures. I had to change my mindset about smiling and now I smile all the time…

There's something in the twinkle of your eyes when you have a bright wide smile. Young people have bright eyes and bright smiles. A new study published in Psychology and Aging showed that when people looked at photos of happy faces, they guessed the age of the person in the photo as younger than in photos of the same person with a neutral or angry expression. Researchers say it's the first study to show that facial expressions have a major impact on the accuracy and bias of age estimates.

Also when you smile it creates creases around the eyes and mouth which for most is temporary and therefore no one can accurately determine whether those lines and creases are temporary or permanent giving you an edge, as the perception is that those are just smile lines. In addition, smiling has been shown to make people look more attractive, which may make them appear younger.

Guessing Age in Photos

In the study, 154 young, middle-aged, and older adults guessed the age of 171 faces of young, middle-aged, and older men and women with various expressions portrayed on a total of 2,052 photographs. Each face displayed either an angry, fearful, disgusted, happy, sad, or a neutral expression.

The results showed that facial expressions had a big effect on the accuracy of age estimates.

Compared with other facial expressions, the age of neutral faces was estimated most accurately. Meanwhile, the age of happy or smiling faces was underestimated by an average of about two years.

So smile your way to a more youthful appearance!

#8 LOL – Laugh Out Loud!!!

Seriously… It's no longer a secret that laughter keeps you young. Researchers studying the process of aging know that laughter improves blood circulation — to the head and to the heart. Laughing is good for you. The scripture in Proverbs even say that "Laughter does the body good like a medicine".

I laugh all the time. There is rarely a day that goes by that I don't have a good belly laugh. A good belly laugh every day improves mood, improves physical health and improves emotional health. Best of all, it's free to everyone.

Here are a couple jokes that might make you LOL:

- "I feel like my body has gotten totally out of shape, so I got my doctor's permission to join a fitness club and start exercising. I decided to take an aerobics class for seniors. I bent, twisted, gyrated, jumped up and down, and perspired for an hour. But, by the time I got my leotards on, the class was over".

- My memory's not as sharp as it used to be. Also, my memory's not as sharp as it used to be.

- As you get older, your secrets are safe with your friends. They can't remember them either.

- I live in my own little world. But it's okay --- they know me here.

- Forget health food. I'm at the age where I need all the preservatives I can get.

- I would be unstoppable, if I could only get started...

- "I am having amnesia, dementia, and I, all at the same time. I think I've forgotten this before . . ."

Remember: You don't stop laughing because you grow old,

You grow old because you stop laughing.

Physical Health Benefits

Laughing heartily and uncontrollably provides a physical release.   Several muscles are exercised including the diaphragm, the abdomen muscles and the shoulders. Blood circulation is increased for all major body organs including the brain. Laughter even provides some exercise for the heart. Increased blood circulation stimulates facial muscles so you might even look better!

Some researchers report that laughter can reduce pain. Increasingly, medical experts use laughter therapy in cancer care and with other chronic illnesses.

When we laugh, stress hormone levels are reduced and levels of healthy hormones are increased. The body's immune system improves with the release of endorphins, those natural 'feel-good' chemicals.

There are so many benefits to laughter that I would need to write a separate book to count them all and if laughing is a struggle for you...'Fake it till you make it'. Researchers say that your body can't distinguish between real or fake laughing. You get the health benefits regardless of whether it is fake or real laughter.

There was a tickle study, yes a tickle study done and here are 12 REAL health benefits to tickling resulting in laughter according to selfgrowth.com...

1.	Blood Circulation produces up to 12% more oxygen and glucose (energy) for body and mind when you smile or laugh often.

2.	Speed of brain functions: up to 15% higher for optimal cognition.

3.	Stress: reduced from mind and body (up to 18% by MRI reading).

4.	Abdominal muscles and digestion strengthened by laughing.

5.	Left and right brain: synchronized and integrated to work together.

6.	Blood pressure lowered up to 10% based on how many smiles & duration of our daily laughing.

7.   Diaphragmatic (deeper) breathing for up to six hours afterward.

8.   Immune System produces a supply of Dopamine – (neurotransmitter) the pleasure hormone.

9.   Attentiveness, heartbeat regularity and pulse rate are improved.

10.   Long-term memory and learning skills enhanced up to 2x (double).

11.   University of Maryland research: protection from stroke and heart attack.

12.   Pain (physical and mental) is reduced up to 50% and your healing rate increases by a surge of Endorphins.

So laugh heartily to stay young and strong!

#9 Stay Away From The Sun

When I was 13 years old, I went on a 1 day field trip to the Island of Tobago with my class. We spent all day on the beach, in and out of the water. Yes it was a whole lot of fun but by the next day I found myself with a wicked sun burn. Back then no one cared about sunblock or sunscreen, plus as a young woman of color, who would have thought I would be susceptible to such a severe burn. Since then I have been very careful about how long and how much exposure I get to direct sunlight.

Ok so not everyone can stay away from the sun, so be safe and use a sunscreen and or sunblock. Using a broadspectrum SPF 30 – 50 daily will prevent skin from ageing prematurely. Upping your SPF protection will make a dramatic difference in how your skin ages. If you will be in the sun all day long at the beach or park, I would suggest layering your sunscreen with a sunblock, why? Because a sunblock, while it provides the best sun protection by providing a wall between your skin and the sun, it only blocks out UVB rays, it doesn't block those UVA rays according to Family Health & Nutrition. So it is essential to also use a sunscreen that pulls double duty for UVA & UVB rays. Tanning oils provide no sun protection so beware.

Here are some quick tips to protect your skin from premature aging from the sun:

- Understand that dark skin can burn just as easily as fair skin, so everyone needs to use sunscreen/sunblock when out in the sun.

- Reapply your sunscreen often if you are going to be in the sun for many hours.

- Understand that layering multiple sunscreen products does not multiply the effect of the sunscreen. Rather which ever product whether it is applied first or second, you will only have the benefit of the highest rated SPF product.

- Clothing can make a huge difference. Wearing White or light colored clothes will increase your sun protection. In addition there are clothes available now with SPF protection built in. If you have kids or work out outdoors a lot, you should look for clothes with SPF protection built in to the fabric.

- This is a great one. Did you know certain foods rich in antioxidants can help prevent your skin from sun damage? Yes there are foods that can protect your body from the inside out. Dark leafy vegetables like Kale, spinach loaded with vitamin C. Red fruit and vegetables like tomatoes, beets, chili peppers have lycopene. Sweet potato, rich in vitamin A. Foods and nuts high in Omega 3's and foods with carotenoids will provide sun protection from the inside out and prevent sun burns.

• You can use oils like Raspberry seed oil, carrot seed oil, wheat germ oil, coconut oil and sesame oil which provide good sun protection but only for short periods of time.

• Protect your eyes with sunglasses.

• Astaxanthin – This is a supplement that is a potent antioxidant derived from Algae and carotenoids. It prevents DNA damage from the sun.

So watch your sun intake & protect your skin!

#10 Create a Daily Skin Care Routine

When I was in High School, about 15 years old, my favorite teacher in her 60's had the most beautiful skin. One day I asked her what her secret was, and she told me that since she was 18 she used Oil of Olay. So, of course, I immediately begged my mom to get me a bottle of Oil of Olay right, what a recommendation! Well sadly it didn't agree with my skin but the lesson I did take away from that conversation was you should take good care of your skin. I went through several skincare routines and tried many lines before I found what worked. It is vitally important that you take the time to care for your skin and find the right products that work for your particular skin type and texture. Consult a specialist if you have to because there are so many choices out there and, I'm sorry to say, that a lot of times it will be a process of trial and error to find the right combination that works for you, that's what I had to do.

Here are some tips that are important for you to follow in your basic skincare regimen:

a.   Incorporate a hydrating Serum – Serums have become extremely popular in the last few years because of its effective delivery system that penetrates further into the layers of skin to affect change. Most of them have a base of hyaluronic acid which holds 1000 times its weight in moisture and helps draw moisture into the skin.

b.   Pay attention to your lips - Soft pillowy lips are a sure sign of youth, but what is it that makes your lips age over time? "As we age, the muscles and tendons that hold our mouths in a pleasant position start to become weak, and our mouths slowly turn down at the corners," says aesthetic dermatologist Whitney Bowe, MD. "A turned-down mouth adds age to the face and makes you appear unhappy or angry even when you're not." A little later I'll introduce a device you can use to help stimulate the muscles in the face, but beyond that, it is incredibly important to exfoliate your lips and keep them moisturized, especially in cold weather and at night. Another tip is to avoid using straws too much because drinking through a straw is similar to smoking for your lips, it can create vertical crease lines along the top of your lips. Smoking however is so much more destructive to your lips because it destroys the collagen that supports the muscles around the lips.

c.   Take the time to properly cleanse your face at night and, yes ladies, that means washing off your makeup at night every night before bed. Your skin absorbs and tries to rejuvenate itself while you sleep, and makeup, if not properly removed, will clog pores and cause more harm if you repeatedly sleep with it on. I don't ever go to bed without a clean moisturized face.

d.   Moisturize entire body especially in winter – I learned this trick a long time ago in my teens, especially in winter I add Vaseline or baby oil gel to my body lotion. That little tip has served me well, because it has kept my skin soft and supple.

e.   Exfoliate - You can slough off dead skin from your face, neck and chest using a natural scrub made of Sea Salt and Sugar, it'll dissolve easily and is not as abrasive as apricot or walnut scrubs that are made from crushed seeds. These types of abrasives are less likely to cause inflammation. Many disagree with me but I gently exfoliate my entire body every single day.

f.   At home spa treatments – Ok this is one I've used in the last few years and I have to admit I'm not as consistent as I should be but I alluded to it earlier when talking about lips. My at home spa is from NuSkin. It delivers microcurrent technology designed to stimulate collagen and tone the skin. This has helped subtly lift areas of my face.

g.   Do NOT EVER sleep in makeup!!! It can clog your pores, and does not give your skin the opportunity to breathe and rejuvenate. I know I said it above but it bears repeating. Too many women sleep in makeup – STOP IT!!!

h.   Lastly, hydrate, hydrate, hydrate!!!

So take good care of all of your skin!

#11 Run for your life

Yes I said in the introduction that this book will not be about diet and exercise because we all already know that those are essential components to a healthy life and longevity. However I felt it necessary to include this tip because for the past 2 years it has helped me tremendously and helped a lot of other people I've shared it with.

For years I was a walker, I would walk about 3 miles about 3-4 times a week. It took me sometimes an hour sometimes less but it was my exercise. On the odd occasion I would go to the gym and run on the treadmill then some weights for an hour. The problem with all of that was that there was no noticeable difference to my body. My weight stayed the same and I wasn't getting any more toned. I found my thighs to still have cellulite and not much muscle tone. No, I wasn't a gym rat doing a gazillion squats and sit ups but so many experts say you should exercise for at least 20 mins to see benefits and there I was doing an hour plus.

Ok, so there were several reasons my exercises weren't yielding the results I wanted. First of all inconsistency, it was a killer. Secondly, the level of intensity was also inconsistent, and thirdly, I didn't really enjoy it.

That all changed after listening to an interview with Tony Robbins where he said every morning he jumps into an ice bath to wake his body up and change its state, I decided that I was going to do something in the mornings to up the ante. So one day instead of walking my usual 3 miles (which by the way took me so long that sometimes weeks would go by before I'd get out again to do it), I decided I would run for as fast as I could for as long as I could without stopping. So I did it around my block which was about ¾ of a mile and took me around 7 minutes to complete. THAT FELT SO GOOD! So I started doing it 4 times a week, and some weeks every day. This has not only changed my life but many other people's lives that I have shared my strategy with. By running 7 minutes, I was able to not only up the intensity of my workout, but I could be so much more consistent because I didn't really have a valid excuse for not setting aside 7 minutes for myself. I noticed that by running, I quickly reshaped and toned my legs and my mid-section. The benefits of the high intensity cardio was amazing. Yes running can be hard on the body, on your knees, joints, and skin, however just 7 minutes 3-4 times a week isn't as hard on the body as running for an hour 3-4 times per week.

So just to clarify I'm not talking about walking or strolling or even jogging, I'm talking about going as fast as you can for as long as you can. Today that same block takes me less than 6 mins to complete. Folks often laugh when I tell them what I do and for how long and ask me why not go a mile, or run longer, well, because I found a formula that works for me and I'm not here to break any records or impress anyone, I just want to be strong and healthy. Before you do any of this, please check with your doctor to make sure you are able to run because the last thing you need is to sustain an injury that will set you back.

I know some of you reading this might say, but Alicia I can't run and I understand that, but the principle behind this is, do what you can do, raise the level of intensity for a shorter period of time and be more consistent.

So if you can, get out and RUN!

#12 Rev up your metabolism

I've always had an active metabolism, but after my 3rd child and a couple of years, I turned 40 and my metabolism took a dive. I knew I needed a kickstart to get it revved up again. So here are some of the things I did, in addition to a couple of those I've already mentioned previously, that helped jumpstart my metabolism.

a.   I lost 15 lbs on a cellular cleanse which detoxed my body. Sounds rough but in actuality it wasn't bad at all. I knew that I had been carrying more weight on my body than I normally did so I committed to a 30 day cleanse which shifted so many things in a positive way in my body and got me jumpstarted again. (To be completely honest, I did 24 of the 30 days, but got the results I needed) . The benefits of the cellular detox meant my body wasn't fighting itself daily to get rid of all the toxins but was running at optimum levels.

b.   Spiced up my life – I love spicy foods, which go along well with my spicy personality, and so continuing to add spice to every meal helps keep my metabolism running well. Statistically it's proven to boost metabolism by 8% - I say we need every little bit of increase we can get.

c.   I chew my food endlessly before swallowing, that helps the digestive process speed up as well.

d.   Drinking more water, (which I will go into more detail in tip #20) as water helps all areas of the body function better.

e.   Drinking tea – Drinking tea has been a part of my life since childhood. It's high in antioxidants and polyphenols which promote good health.

f.   Eating smaller meals many times a day. I eat small meals throughout the day, some researchers say it doesn't do anything for your metabolism, however, I noticed that for me, I don't get that sluggish feeling when I just maintain a fueled body instead of eating a huge meal that I need to take a nap afterwards from. I would rather eat small portions of real food 5 times a day than eat 3 big meals and snack junk in between.

g.   Eating Breakfast especially high in protein. Ok I have always been a big proponent of eating breakfast but since doing my cleanse I mentioned earlier, I have a protein shake for breakfast loaded with fruits. That is my breakfast and it really holds me well for the entire morning. If I don't have a shake I have eggs or Sardines but something that is filled with protein because studies have shown that protein makes your body exert more energy in order to digest it therefore helping you burn more.

h.   Stop eating after a certain time at night. I have basically stopped eating after 7:00 pm. Occasionally I end up eating later but that's just once in a while. It has really helped keep my weight in check. When I was younger though, I could eat anything at any time, including a huge meal right before bed and it never affected me. But after 40, that no longer worked, it slowed my metabolism way down and I began gaining weight. Now that I have adopted this new schedule, I have to be so disciplined. So after 7:00

pm, no food, and no snacks, (Ok maybe sometimes I snack a little, lol).

i. I run instead of walk. Running for me has really helped kick start my day and that's how I use and burn energy. There's more on how and when I run in tip #11.

So rev up that Metabolism!

#13 Clothes make the man/woman

As a style expert I am often asked "Am I too old to wear..."

Ok there are some styles you should avoid as you age but the bigger concern is fit not style. Understanding your body Type will go a long way in making you look younger because when you find what fits your body and the style that works best for your body type, no matter what it is, it will make you look younger.

One of your first priorities in dressing your body is to determine your goal. What are you searching for?

- A Balanced body

- Slimming

- Volume

- Accentuate your curves/ Particular body parts

- Create shape

Determine where you are so you can create a plan for where you want to be...

Body type – Finding out your vertical and horizontal body type is the first step to dressing for success. Why, because understanding how clothes fit your body and what flatters and what detracts will allow you to always look your best. There are clothes that can make you look streamlined and compliment you in all the right ways. When your clothes fit your body, you can wear many different styles even things you think might be too young for you to wear.

<u>Determining your horizontal body type:</u>

Use a tape measure and measure your bust line, waist line and your hip at the widest point. Once you have those numbers you can determine your horizontal body.

Inverted triangle – Shoulders and/or bust line measures more than your waist and hips.

Rectangle – There is very little difference between your 3 key areas.

Apple or round – If your waist or mid-section measures more than your hips and sometimes bust.

Pear or triangle – Hips measure more than the bust and waist.

Hourglass – Bust and hip measure close and waist measures less than both.

Vertical Body Type:

This determines your vertical proportions, if you have a long torso, short waist, long waist, if you are petite, regular or tall. Take your tape measure and place it in the hollow between your collar bone, then measure the distance between there and the base of your crotch. Find your waist, if it measures half the distance then you have a balanced torso, if the distance between the hollow in the collar bone and natural waist is less than the waist to below the crotch, then you are short waisted, and will typically have longer legs. Similarly if the distance between the hollow and your waist is longer than the waist to crotch, then you have a long torso and typically shorter legs.

Weight – Sometimes we are not at our ideal weight. I understand that, because I was there, but that doesn't mean while you are working on it, you can't still wear clothes that fit your body correctly. Don't stay unhappy or dissatisfied if you are not where you want to be, do something about it, because carrying extra weight on your body ages you.

Size – I always tell my clients not to get hung up on sizes. The reason is if you are way too invested in the size of your clothes instead of the fit, you could find yourself wearing something that doesn't fit you right. You see sizes aren't standardized - some designers run smaller in their sizes while others run larger, my suggestion is to always try things on to find the best fit for your clothes.

Here are a couple tips to help you achieve your goal:

- Slimming – Wear a totally monochromatic look from head to toe. Use vertical lines or Chevron patterns in clothing or a long sweater open in the middle to draw the eye up and down.

- Create volume – Use horizontal or diagonal lines, large prints, patterns, bright colors.

- Accentuate or create shape – Color blocking can create the shape you want along with pattern.

- If you have a short waist avoid midriffs and high waist pants/skirts. If you have a long waist, avoid hipster pants/skirts.

So find the style that best suit your body type and make sure you have the best fit!

#14 Foods & Supplements that Build & Improve Collagen.

Most of my life I have taken fish oil capsules, I believe that along with flaxseed this has helped my skin looking young. Other foods and supplements you should have in your diet which I enjoy tremendously are foods rich in Vitamin C, Retinoids, peptides and Omega 3. I also eat high proteins from sources like peanuts, eggs, fish (especially Salmon), lentils, beef, and chicken. Benefits of taking 1,000 Mil of Fish Oil per day either from Krill oil or other forms of fish oil can heal dry, rough skin and ultimately these essential fats are a key component of the lubricating layer that keeps skin supple.

Here are 11 collagen boosting foods to add to your shopping list

1.   Fish rich in Omega 3 fatty acids like Tuna and Salmon.

2.   Red vegetables and fruits like tomatoes, chili peppers and beets. They are high in antioxidants and lycopene provides sun protection from the inside and increases collagen.

3.   Dark green vegetables like Kale and spinach. They are high in vitamin C and rev up metabolism.

4.   Orange vegetables like carrots and sweet potatoes are rich in vitamin A which helps restore and regenerate.

5.   Berries scavenge free radicals while simultaneously building collagen.

6.   Soy contains a plant hormone that blocks enzymes that age the skin.

7.   White tea prevents enzyme activity that breaks down collagen.

8.   Citrus, again high in vitamin C aids in boosting collagen both topically and internally.

9.   High protein foods like meat and nuts are the building blocks for collagen.

10.   Garlic contains sulfur necessary for collagen production and lipoic acid.

11.   Oysters contain zinc, vitamins, B12 and minerals that aid in collagen production.

So eat to boost your collagen!

#15 Hair Cut &/ or Color

There is so much debate about whether to gray or not to gray... Well I have lots and lots of gray hair, it's hereditary, but I am not about to grow it out, nope not yet at all. Why? Because unless the gray is all over and covers 80% to 90% of your head, which can look really cool, gray roots can age you prematurely. Personally I prefer to color them and not look like a skunk. Now there will come a point where coloring them will not look natural anymore, believe me when I say, I'll cross that bridge when I get there! Just a quick note about hair color unless your goal is for your hair color to look unnatural, like purple, orange, green, pink etc, do not continue to color your hair beyond the point where it can look natural.

Listen having your hair just 'blah' does nothing for you. Consult with a stylist and get a cut that flatters your face. I've heard that women over 40 shouldn't have long hair, well that's a bunch of baloney. They definitely can but it needs to be healthy, shiny and have a modern feel to it.

So cut, color and style your hair!

#16 Take Care of Neck, Chest, Elbows and Hands.

There are certain areas of the body that show age more than others and those areas are often neglected. Neck, décolleté, or chest, elbow and hands are often overlooked. I have made it my business to properly take good care of those areas because as we age, our skin gets thinner and unless you keep these areas well moisturized they can show even faster.

Quick tips for taking care of these important but sometimes neglected areas:

1.   Use sunscreen on your neck and chest if you will be out in the sun and have them exposed.

2.   When moisturizing your face, bring it all the way down to your neck. Use a moisturizer with Retinol A to reduce fine lines and age spots.

3.   Always carry hand lotion in your purse. Immediately apply lotion to hands after washing. This will help your hands stay soft and supple. Also don't leave out those elbows. So many times elbows are neglected until they start to look dry and scaly. Using a firming cream can also help those elbows stay looking younger.

So take good care of your neck, elbows, décolleté, and hands! Moisturize, moisturize, moisturize!

#17 Using Effective Makeup Techniques

Being a professional Makeup Artist has helped me in this area, so here are some basic tips that can help you. As we age, our skin changes in color, texture and tone. Some develop dark circles, fine lines, age spots, adult acne, or skin discoloration due to hyperpigmentation. It becomes even more important to learn how to color correct to get the right coverage when wearing makeup. The skin on your face like the rest of your body fall victim to gravity and many things that were once in one location have unfortunately shifted. It's a cruel, cruel joke and many run out and seek botox, laser treatments or fillers to try to turn back the clock.

There is absolutely nothing wrong with seeking these treatments, but do your research carefully before choosing someone to work with. Be your own advocate and get recommendations for those you trust and don't go based on price, this is not the time to be cheap.

However, if you're like me and would rather not have procedures done, (I'm a chicken) learning a few simple makeup techniques can help create the look you want.

Your makeup routine will have to change. What worked for you in your 20's is not going to work the same in your 40's and beyond especially if you are dealing with any of the above mentioned issues. Here are my simple tips to help you create a more youthful appearance.

1.   Skin discoloration and Hyper-pigmentation.

a.   It is essential to color correct before applying foundation. If you have rosacea or redness in your skin, you'll need a yellow or green base to first

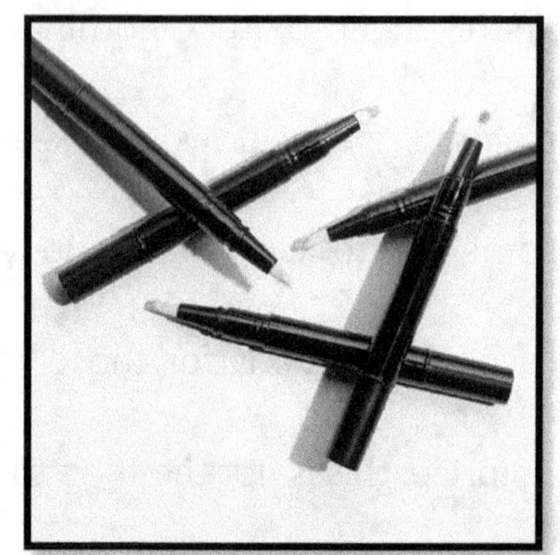

neutralize the red and bring balance to the skin and restore your radiance. For brown or dark spots, including under eye circles you would need an orange, apricot, peachy or red base depending on how deep the discoloration is. Apply the color corrector, set it with a translucent powder then apply the foundation.

b.   Use a foundation that has buildable coverage. A medium coverage foundation allows you to apply your foundation without a heavy cakey look which ages you. You can build coverage just where you need it.

2.   Contouring/highlighting: It's important to understand the structure of your face. Like I said earlier, as we age the location of some of your features may have shifted south so understanding how to create the illusion of higher cheekbones, bigger eyes and a chiseled jawline can go a long way to bringing back your youth.

3.   Thicker eyebrows: As we age eyebrows can become thinner, by shaping and filling in your brows you can achieve a much more youthful look. It also helps when you use a brow pen to cover any gray hair.

4.   Create eye looks that lift: Sometimes your eyes become hooded or begin to turn downward in the corners.

a.   If hooding occurs and you do not want to have an eyelift because it is mild, you can use this simple trick, highlight the lid of your eye with a shadow that pops, then create a crease with a darker flat matte shade and apply it from the crease to the brow bone but pull the color a little above where the brow bone begins. Use a shadow that does not have a high shimmer to highlight the brow bone. Then blend to soften the colors.

b.   If your eyes begin to turn down at the outer corner, the simple fix for that is to apply your eyeliner differently. Instead of following the eye line with the liner exactly, start lining from the inner corner and when you come 2/3rds of the way past the pupil begin to draw the line slightly upward, then stop just beyond the corner of your eyes. Note, this is not a cateye look.

A lot of these techniques will require practice and can get you the look you want.

So use makeup techniques that bring out your inner glow!

#18 Avoid Alcohol

While a lot of studies tout the benefits of certain Alcoholic beverages like Wine, I've never really been a big fan of any kind of adult beverage, not since I was in my late teens and tried it. There was really nothing I enjoyed about drinking, not the taste or the way it made me feel, so after just a couple tries I figured it was just one of those things I wouldn't ever indulge in.

So how has not drinking alcohol been beneficial to me? Well for one, alcohol is very dehydrating to the system and as we age we need as much hydration as possible so unless you drink lots of water to compensate for the dehydrating effects of the alcohol your skin will show the signs of dehydration from the inside out. While alcohol itself won't *cause* cellulite, alcohol constricts blood vessels in the skin, which makes cellulite worse. What you may not know too is that alcohol promotes fluid retention and increases fat deposits in areas like your thighs, arms, abdomen and glutes.

Not to mention the fact that alcohol is just all "empty calories" that can lead to weight gain and doesn't provide any nutritional benefits whatsoever.

So if you can, you should avoid alcohol but if you choose to drink, then make sure you hydrate, hydrate, hydrate, your skin will thank you for it!

#19 – No Smoking

My encounter with smoking was as short lived as my encounter with alcohol. I tried it as a teen and decided it was definitely NOT for me.

Ok, ok yes there are many reasons NOT to smoke, and yes I'm going to add one more. Smoking ages you. Here are some of the ways smoking ages you prematurely.

1.   Cellulite, yes it can increase cellulite and here's how. Cigarette smoke can reduce blood vessel flow, which will weaken and disrupt the formation of collagen. That causes the connective tissue to stretch, weaken, and become damaged more easily. As a result, more underlying fat—aka cellulite—will show through.

2.   The weakening of collagen and elastin will affect the skin causing it to sag faster especially in your face. Tell tail

signs are, deep wrinkles and lines, unusually loose skin and puffy under eyes, jowls around the jawline and lips that have deep vertical lines all around the edges called the smokers pucker.

3.	Smoking destroys your teeth, they become discolored and damaged.

4.	Because it deprives the skin of oxygen, age spots are darker and lips become discolored.

5.	Smoking also damages the hair follicles causing hair loss.

So don't smoke and avoid second hand smoke!

#20 – Drink Lots of Water

I am a water drinker… yes I drink water more than anything else. I still think I don't drink enough but I am a big advocate of water drinking. When I go out with friends to 'happy hour' I used to get teased because while others were ordering cocktails I would always order water, I finally said to my critics that I choose to eat my calories not drink empty ones. My Pastor, Stan Moore Sr. wrote an entire book on the health benefits of drinking water. Water is the main component in the composition of our bodies in fact it's up to 2/3 of our bodies so it would stand to reason that we need water to survive and thrive. The benefits increase exponentially when that water is alkaline.

Here are some of the many benefits to drinking water.

1.   Healthy hydrated skin. Your skin will be supple and radiant which not only looks youthful but also stays youthful.

2.   It relieves fatigue; dehydration causes you to feel sluggish and fatigued. One way to be more youthful is to have lots and lots of energy.

3.   Helps in digestion, foods can easily be digested and it will allow nutrients to be properly absorbed.

4.   Water flushes your body of toxins and as stated before, when you are able to reduce the toxicity in your system, your body functions more optimally.

5.   There can also be weight loss benefits to adequate water consumption.

6.   Drinking water can also improve your mood. Happy people are also perceived as younger.

So drink water to improve your health!

#21 – Love Yourself

It is absolutely vital to do things to love yourself; especially as women. We are the nurturers in our families and take care of everyone else's needs before our own. This is usually to our detriment. Remember I was a flight attendant and before every flight we would tell the passengers with children to place the mask on their own face before assisting others, yet in real life, we do the opposite because it feels selfish to take care of your needs. STOP that right now. I love music and love to dance, I can't always go out to dance but that doesn't stop me from turning the music up and dancing wild and crazy like no one is watching... My kids are usually watching though totally mortified. So get a massage if you like that, get your nails done, find something that nurtures you and do it.

Meditation, is another great way to love yourself. My prayer time is my meditation time. I enjoy reading my bible and praying, sometimes quietly and sometimes out loud, but that is my time.

Get enough sleep. Sleep is so vital to your health and the ability of your body to rejuvenate itself. It's important to get good quality sleep, because it releases growth hormone and melatonin both of which have major anti-aging benefits.

Gratitude has to be a part of your routine in loving yourself. Take the time to find things you are thankful for. Being thankful takes your mind off of the negative things in your life and allows you to be happier, again happier people look are younger.

This final tip is not one I personally have a challenge with but many of my friends are dealing with this and it is hormonal imbalance. Bioidentical hormones or compounding hormones have changed women's lives. So what are bioidentical hormones, I am not a doctor but according to many of my contacts that are obgyn's and specialize in identifying women with the symptoms that indicate hormonal imbalance, bioidentical hormones are synthesized in a lab with the exact molecular match to those made naturally in the body (with limited to no side effects). Many women experience fatigue, fuzziness, lack of clarity, weight gain and low libido but have no idea what's going on in their bodies. From what I understand, a typical examination won't indicate the deficiencies and many doctors wouldn't recommend bioidenticals for you because either they have no experience with it or they really don't know about it. So before you give up or feel discouraged, find a doctor that specializes in bioidentical hormone therapy to see if you are a candidate. I've had friends whose lives have absolutely transformed in just a couple of days on these hormones. Be your best advocate of your health, if you don't feel like yourself, do some research and get it checked out.

So, find multiple ways to love yourself!

Aging Gracefully – Leilla Blackwell

The Fountain of Youth can be seen as a metaphor for the exhilarating flow of energy that accompanies the intensity of the supercharged, wet, gushing female

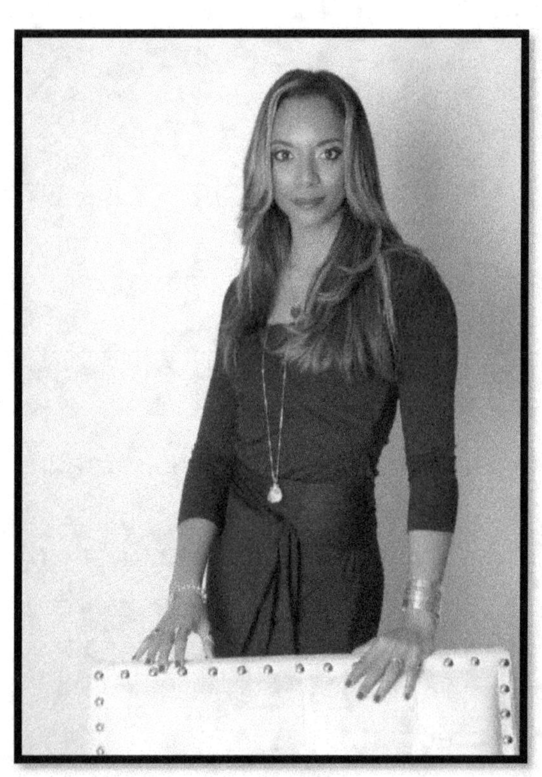

orgasm. As women, we are blessed to have access to health and longevity through pleasure. The even greater gift is that the experience of orgasm is heightened with the right partner, cultivating meaningful human connections that foster extended satisfaction, happiness and joy throughout different areas of our lives. Orgasm is nature's medicine for all aspects of aging, including emotional health, mental clarity, efficiency of internal body systems, bone density and muscular functioning, and external beauty and radiance. It generates excellence from the inside out.

We can start to understand the real significance of orgasm, by taking a closer look at its impact on stress, which is widely known to accelerate aging. Stress is notorious for causing disease, such as heart disease, high blood pressure, and even certain forms of cancer, as well as unhealthy relationships with food, alcohol and drugs, including prescription medications. Stress interferes with basic functions like digestion, sleep and metabolism. Stress affects our posture, body movements and facial expressions. It also directly affects our relationships with co-workers, family, friends, children, and intimate partners. There begins the vicious cycle of chronic stress, because as these systems break down, stress snowballs. Over time, chronic stress leads to an excess of free radicals in the body, which, in addition to wrinkles on the outside, ages us at the cellular DNA level and can be linked to thyroid burnout, Parkinson's, Alzheimer's and dementia. The stress hormone, cortisol, is largely responsible for the biological repercussions of mental and emotional stress. The primary hormone released through the intensely pleasurable experience of orgasm is oxytocin, which directly lowers cortisol levels and combats stress.

Oxytocin is also known as the "love hormone." It cuts down the stress response and anxiety that tend to interfere with relationships, while simultaneously fostering human connections, trust, secure bonding and intimacy; creating a new snowball effect of love, connectedness, and more meaningful intimate relationships. Greater intimacy contributes to the potential for orgasmic experiences and a new flood of oxytocin.

An increased level of oxytocin balances estrogen production. Estrogen increases a woman's femininity, including breast volume, wider hips and smaller waist (that sexy hourglass shape), better sex drive and sexual responsiveness, and the mothering instinct. Lower levels of estrogen are associated with dry sagging skin, joint pain, excess facial hair, fatigue and mental fog; all signs of aging.

Oxytocin isn't the only hormone directly impacted by orgasm. A rush of all the happy hormones, like serotonin, dopamine and endorphins, can be

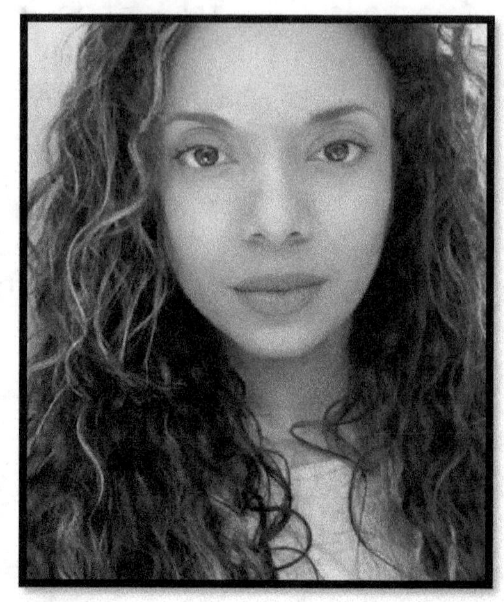

increased in women and men through orgasm. Serotonin helps us feel significant and content, dopamine supplies motivation, and endorphins reduce pain and anxiety while giving us a sense of aliveness. We all know when we see someone filled to overflowing with love and happiness, who seems motivated, fully alive and at ease in their skin, they come across as youthful.

As a woman in her mid-forties, I see youth as an inside job. I live in a general state of openness, in the flow of life. Some people may even call me naïve, or see me as a "Pollyanna" type. It can be easy to mistake an accepting, peaceful, youthful spirit for an oblivious mentality. While I am filled with bliss, gratefully it doesn't stem from ignorance. Finding a state of happiness in a world filled with opportunities for misery can seem like an impossible feat.

Throughout my adult life, I have enjoyed loving, lasting relationships, including with my husband of over 20 years, our children, family, friends and my profession. That doesn't mean I don't experience stress from those same relationships. It does mean that a lifestyle of healthy eating, exercise, prayer, meditation, tons of laughter, gratitude and appreciation for the full breadth and depth of the human experience, punctuated by an abundant, active, multi-orgasmic sex life, helps me counter life's stressors. I couldn't say for sure which came first, because it's all part of an integrated lifestyle. If I am viewed as youthful, it stems from a spirit of aliveness, which for me is linked to this delicious cocktail that I wouldn't attempt to alter.

Youth in your 60's - Connie Hertz

I'm Connie Hertz and I'm happy to share with you many things I have done to remain 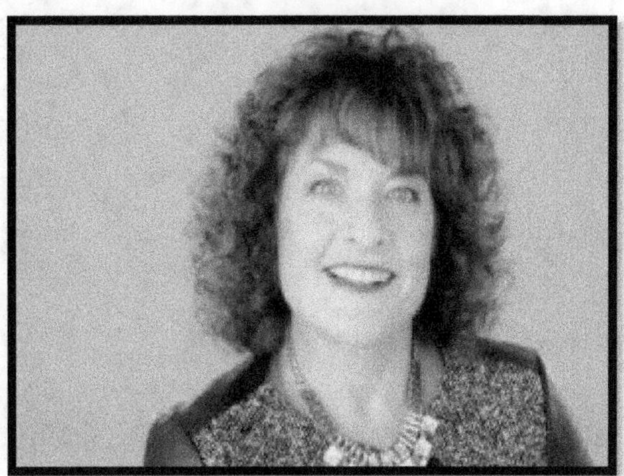 youthful, energetic and looking younger than my 62 years.

As I read Alicia's book with her tips on staying younger longer, I have consciously done the majority of her tips on a regular basis.

I am 62 years young and I think of myself as still being in my early 30's!

In 1974 I took my first personal growth class that taught me about meditation and a positive mindset. I have been practicing on a very regular basis meditation and also studying and learning about the importance of a positive attitude and mindset in order to create a life you love.

I also have been taking great supplements each day and I'm careful about what food I eat. Thus never being overweight as Alicia covers in her tips.

I studied health and nutrition along with nursing back in 1974 as well. I became an oncology nurse back in the 1970's and now I'm a certified life coach.

As Alicia talks about how important it is to eat healthy and to drink lots of water in relation to looking and feeling younger, I know these things plus exercising at least 4 days every week, mixing it up with cardio and weight training for over 35 years now, have kept me healthy, fit and looking and feeling more youthful.

Alicia talks about in one of her tips taking care of your teeth. I agree this is something that I adopted now close to 40 years ago and I never go a night without flossing my teeth and using a water pik!

As far as skin care, I have been using wonderful anti-aging skin care for many years and I never go to sleep without taking off my makeup and applying my serum's and lotions. Another thing I think that goes along with having a positive mindset and attitude is consciously continuing to grow and learn. I have written in a daily gratitude journal and I read inspiring readings and pray every morning, for many years now too. No matter where I'm at, I make time to do my personal practices every day.

I also have written a weekly blog called "Sharing From My Heart" for just over 4 years. This gives me a chance to share with others, my wisdom I have learned for the last 62 years, including times of pain and sorrow and now living in JOY more of my present moments than not.

So, I would say being consistent with these practices and tips I have shared and Alicia has shared, is key to making them a part of your life. I would caution you to take it slowly as you add in each new practice and be gentle with yourself!

I know as a life coach, that as people start doing new things and too many of them at once, they give up too soon because they get discouraged with themselves. So take it all one or two new things at a time and as you've mastered them and they become part of your daily life, then you can add in another one or two more new practices.

Loving yourself as Alicia says is very important. So pay attention to what you're feeling and saying to yourself every day. Take deep breaths and slow down and stop living on auto-pilot. Stop to appreciate people and things in your life. As you do, you'll find yourself smiling more and living more in joy more of your present moments than you ever have.

All of these things keep you looking and feeling young, alive and vibrant! Here's to your youthfulness and living in joy!

Have Faith – Laure Carter

For the first part of my life I was a care-free, adventurous young woman. I followed my intuition about places and people and met the 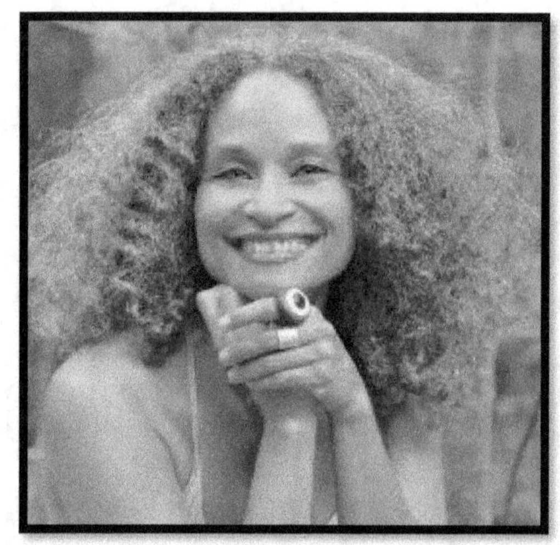 most interesting people and found myself in some of the most gorgeous places in the world, Cairo, Chang Mai, Marrakech...

And then one day I lost my trust in life, I'm not quite sure how that exactly happened but I did and I started struggling and worrying. The moment that happened I aged, worrying lines started showing on my brow, my jaw tightened giving me this hard look.

I began to think that life was hard and that I was not safe and I started wanting to control it.

Guess what? The more I tried to control it, the more out of control it felt! And the older and heavier I felt inside.

I spent almost twenty years worrying about everything, money, relationships, my health, my work.

Did worrying make things better, safer? Of course not! My body began to break down and I experienced chronic back pain while I was teaching people about getting out of pain in my yoga studio.

My mind was filled with anxiety and most nights I would wake up in the middle of the night scared to death for no reason, while I was teaching my students how to meditate.

I was in my early forties and looked fifty.

Everything came to a tipping point when arriving at Indira Gandhi airport in New Delhi and got into a taxi, bam! Into a car accident.

At that moment I could either go into a frenzy in a strange country or I could just let go and how do they say again? Let God.

And I decided to let go!

And I let go of wanting to control. I let go of wanting to struggle. I let go of wanting to worry and be afraid.

And the more I let go, the lighter I felt.

The more I let go, the safer I felt in a long time, because I started to see that at every moment, Life always, always gives me what I need.

The more I let go, the more joyful I felt, because I felt free!

And today, I can tell you that the way to look and feel youthful is to let down the struggle and release the need to control and have faith.

Yes, eating well matters, exercising matters, living your purpose matters, and these things become easier to integrate in your life when you have faith.

Faith is my youth elixir.

Because of faith, I smile easily and laugh heartily, I say yes to the unknown, I trust myself and I trust other people, I feel light and free, I feel the confidence of youth that when I jump I will be caught.

Healthy, Sexy and inspired after Menopause – Angelika Christie

My mother decided to leave her body in her sleep after enjoying the 1938 class reunion with only 10 remaining classmates who she declared old and fragile.

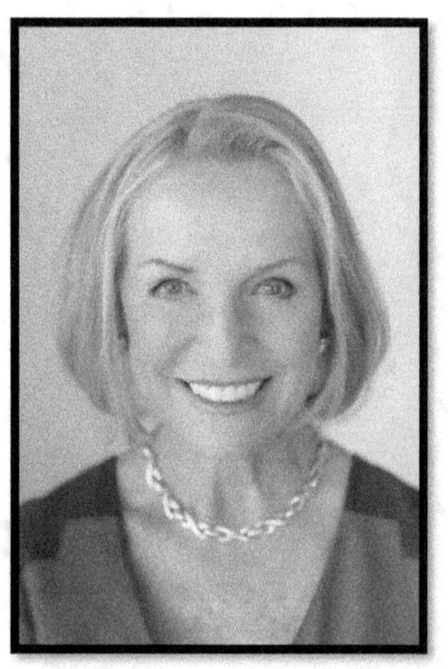

She was quite the opposite, a child-like goddess filled with imagination, creativity, playfulness and beauty. She lived her highest potential creating exceptional paintings and high fashion collections. My mother exuded energy and magnetism; she frequently attracted younger men and women who adored her and tried to be around her as much as possible, even in her eighties! I know that I took her for granted--she was my Mom. There were 3 things she did that I still remember vividly:

1. She kept her slender figure despite her healthy appetite. What I'm saying here is that she could eat 5 course meals!! And add desert. And add wines. And then have a second helping! I never forget how she explained her resilience to any expected digestive troubles with certain foods that I could not eat without bloating or a stomach ache. My mother would say: 'I just talk to my inner Alchemist to deal with it, and he does."

2. My mother also declared that 'not possible' does not exist, but that 'EVERYTHING is possible'. Period!

3. I still hear her voice declaring: Angelika the most important duty in your life is to yourself; make your health and beauty number one.

I wish my mother had shared with me all or at least some of her secrets to staying so young. Also about some of her challenges... but she never talked about aging. Ever.

I guess it did not exist to her.

So why am I using so much space here talking about my mother?

She knew how to be magnetic, because she took delight in herself. She was enthusiastic by experiencing each day anew. She was loving because she only saw the best in everybody. And she was non-judgmental because she was open to being surprised.

My mother demonstrated that being Ageless is more of an Attitude rather than a condition. I learned from that, and you can too.

Now let me share with you my secrets to staying healthy, sexy, and inspired.

All of us desire a healthy physical body, a brilliant mind, sound emotions and discovering our true gifts and abilities and what to do with them. The greatest adventure of your life is Self-Discovery and Self-Realization.

Body/Mind connection:

Remember that your body is your responsibility alone. Embrace this truth with awe for the creator who has designed your body in a way that it takes care of itself as long as you give it the minimum building blocks and don't mess up too badly. That's an awesome power to behold; don't you think so? In other words, your body says YES to everything you think, feel and do. It's like your miniature

Universe. Most of us are unaware of what we tell our bodies.

You may have heard that the Universe doesn't respond to negations. It

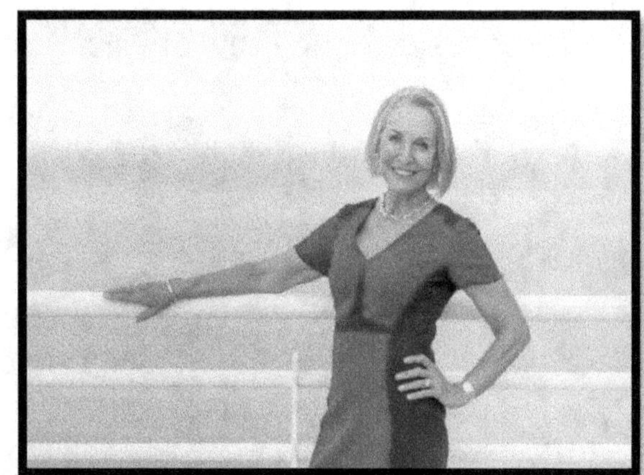

simply gets the command without the "don't". "I don't want to get cancer" and "I don't want to be poor" simply translates "I want to have cancer"… "be poor." That's quite shocking, yes? Check yourself in your thoughts and what you say, and become aware how often you use: "I don't want" then immediately cancel that thought and declare what you want.

If you think that this has little to do with how to stay young, you want to reconsider and spend some time practicing what you want to see manifested in your body and in your life. It starts with how you think and how you feel and what you declare. It sends out a frequency that goes out to find what is in resonance and starts to manifest just that for you.

There is so much more to say about that, and how this truth alone changed everything for the better in my life, even created miracles. If you want to know more about his and the other points that follow from here, let's connect. Pick a time on my online calendar http://www.vcita.com/v/angelikachristie/online_scheduling and get my insight to your questions in a free consultation.

Of course, you know about the basics for health, energy and longevity, which are

- Detox

- Rest

- Sunshine

- Attitude

- Food

- Exercise

They are easy to remember as D.R.S.A.F.E (Dr. Safe) and it represents 1 of 5 Pillars that are essential to your greatest health success. I also believe that due to higher stress levels, pollution, radiation, and poorer food quality, naturally derived and proven effective supplements are necessary as we age.

That's a whole chapter by itself, and as a trained Naturopath and Anti- Aging Specialist I make myself available to discuss your needs on a personal call that you can schedule using the link to my online calendar.

Let me just point out two supplements that I would never miss and nor should you!

They are: Probiotics and Magnesium (both in High Grade Quality). I want to also share some tips that keep me fit, energetic, sexy and inspired.

If you want to:

1.   Look great

2.   Feel great

3.   Be Self Confident

4.   Design great Relationships

5.   Receive Abundance

Due to limited space here, I will be brief yet hope to stimulate your imagination of what is possible for you, and inspire you to try out some of my tips.

Decide to let go of the following:

- Worry (Nothing gets accomplished)

- Rushing (Never necessary, but dangerous)

- Overwhelm (Breathe and focus on one thing at the time)

- Distractions (Turn electronic notifications off and do the most important tasks)

- Judgments (Narrows your ability to find creative solutions)

- Bad Relationships (Say NO and love yourself free)

- Bad Habits (they stand in your way of having what you want.)

Want to know my secret sauce to looking great now and until the day I close my eyes to this world? We have only space for 2 ingredients.

1.   Short and Intense

As a former short distance runner, and Marathon runner after 40, you would think that I recommend running or jogging. NO! NO! NO! Don't do it; there is no health benefit, but rather a health risk associated with running and jogging. Our bodies are not designed to run for long distances, or jog each day at the same speed.   Those (wrongly recommended) habits will wear down you joints make you heart attack prone and shrink your lungs. Really? Yes, REALLY!

What is most important is:

- Your muscle tone

- Your joint and tissue flexibility

- Your ability to calm down your racing heart

- Keeping or expanding your lung capacity

I use my body weight for short and intense 5-8 Minute workouts, twice a day. My heart pounds and I'm panting. My metabolism soars throughout the day, burning food calories for energy rather than depositing fat for storage.

I walk the beach for enjoyment of nature, meditation, and creative downloads. I feel happiest right there each morning. I feel the sun's benefits through my skin and soak up the beneficial negative ions through the soles of my feet.

I feel energized in no time. For other benefits and fun I do really fast step repetitions for 20-30 seconds a few times and often sing out of joyful gratitude to God whom I feel within and everywhere outside me.

If I want to add a bit of intensity, I visualize and separate internal and external muscle groups, which I consciously contract, hold and release. This is not only beneficial for the pelvis floor and abdominal muscle toning, but it's also fun to experience your control over your body. Yep, give commands for your body to follow; real nice Power Trip!

2.   Long and Slow

The long and slow is just as important, since it brings awareness to your mind and flexibility to your body. I used to teach Yoga and Meditation. From my decades of practices, I developed a gentle and easy Yoga routine that I call: "Breath of Peace Yoga" which I practice wherever and whenever I desire, including the ocean the pool, the beach, on a lounge chair, and even in bed. (If you are interested, find out more by contacting me.) The long, slow stretch and breath are powerful and effective for vitality and longevity while keeping your body slender, elongated, elegant, and sexy.

Would love to continue our conversation, but ran out of allowed space here.

Let me close with the most profound realization of my 70+ years of lived experience:

There's only you that will never leave you.

There's only you that knows what's best for you.

There's only you that has the power to create real magic for you.

There's only you who can love you like nobody else.

There's only you who has everything inside to create your unique life.

Consider "Heroic Self Love" as the Master Key to your happy and a prosperous life.

As my gift, I share a powerful tool that calms and clears your mind. Ask by email for my "Focused Hand Meditation." (Video, Audio or PDF) to. Info@angelikachristie.com Subject line: Hand Meditation

Conclusion

I know these 21+ tips I have given you been really simple and that's me super simple. I try my best not to complicate things but to enjoy the simplicity in life and do things that bring me joy. I will encourage you to not overlook it's practicality but instead the benefits.

I have found that society has become so very obsessed with youth, 20 year olds are being encouraged to have botox as a preventative measure against the signs of aging which is so ridiculous to me. Instead of teaching them how to eat healthy and take care of themselves and love themselves no matter what. We have forgotten how to appreciate every moment in life and choose to lie about our age. I meet so many women that do that. I have never lied about my age, because to do that in my opinion, denies all the great and yes sometimes not so great moments that have shaped my life and made me who I am today.

I hope you can look at these 21+ tips and see how you can incorporate some of them into your life and hopefully you will see some benefits as I have.

Resources

Dr. Caroline Leaf - http://drleaf.com/

Dr. Hans Jenny -

http://www.bibliotecapleyades.net/ciencia/ciencia_cymatic

s06.htm

Married with Children -

https://www.youtube.com/watch?v=DikpddPf79g

Dr. Ellen Langer (Mindfulness Institute) -

http://langermindfulnessinstitute.com/portfolio-item/can-

your-mental-attitude-reverse-the-effects-of-aging/

Smile study -

http://www.webmd.com/beauty/aging/20111111/smiling-

makes-you-look-younger

Laughing - http://bottomlinehealth.com/even-a-fake-laugh-

will-do/

Difference between sunscreen & sunblock -

http://oncosec.com/sunscreen-vs-sunblock-whats-the-

difference/

At Home Spa Kit -

https://www.nuskin.com/content/nuskin/en_US/products/shop/shop_all/spa_systems.html

Cellular Cleanse & protein shake – Contact me Alicia@aliciacouri.com for details.

Bioidentical Hormones -

https://gastrolyte.com.au/dehydration/dehydration-and-alcohol/